A History

of *Nursing*

A History *of* Nursing

Poetry by ANNE WEBSTER

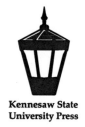

Kennesaw State
University Press

Kennesaw State University Press
Kennesaw State University
Building 27, Suite 220, Mailbox 2701
1000 Chastain Road
Kennesaw, GA 30144

Cathleen Salsburg, Editor & Production Editor
Shirley Parker-Cordell, Senior Administrative Specialist
Holly S. Miller, Book & Cover Design, Production Supervisor
Melissa Stiers, Production Assistant

Library of Congress Cataloging-in-Publication Data

Webster, Anne, 1940-
A History of Nursing / by Anne Webster.
    p. cm.
ISBN-13: 978-1-933483-17-7
1. Nursing--Poetry. 2. Nurses--Poetry. I. Title.
PS3623.E3955H57 2007
811'.6--dc22
                                2007037858

Printed in the United States of America
10 9 8 7 6 5 4 3 2

For Larry, my rock.

And with gratitude to:
my sister Rosemary Daniell, a brilliant writer and teacher, for her role in nurturing my writing; the Atlanta Zona Rosa writing workshop; and the members of the Midtown Writers Group, all of whom have given generously of their support, time, and expertise.

Contents

viii

Four

Five

One

Stuff I Learned in Nursing School

to live in a tiny room with two other girls,
to drink red wine, Cuba libres,
to smoke cigarettes,
to say all the forbidden words:
goddamn, hellfire, fuck, shit,
to French inhale, French kiss—

to swab down eight bodies, make eight beds
at a fast trot, dizzy from not enough sleep
the head nurse yelling like a drill sergeant
before running off to three hours of class,
to learn how to poke needles
in oranges, in my roommate—
which hole for the enema, which for the catheter,
to stand when some asshole doctor
ambles in, all hands—like the one
we call Molest Me Gillespie—
to kiss some intern, me all over him,
like a tabby cat on fire,
then night duty, helping to catch
greasy babies, the gush of blood
missing the bucket, I have to swab
along with clots on forceps—
to keep arm distance from old men's
pinching paws, to flip the sheet
over a show-off's wrinkled weenie,
to scrub for surgery, holding
my hands like the holy mother,
to duck when I hand some
hungover surgeon
the wrong instrument
and the whole tray comes flying at me,
to stifle gags at clouds of stink,
wiping shit-ooze from a withered butt,
or cleaning a bubbly mass,
cancer that used to be pink skin,
to hold my face flat,
even smile and pat an arm
while I'm screaming inside
at guts throbbing in an open belly,
to have some MD come at me

mad dog crazy, snarling,
mouth foaming
when his patient goes bad,
for the whole world to treat me
like a retard maid
when I've just watched
someone's father die,
all of the above my ticket
to punching a time clock
at a job that gives me
a bad back, varicose veins,
work that makes friends think
that they can say any damn thing
about their bodies or their bowels,
that I really want to see
their hairy surgery scars,
and, yes, to have a new patient say,
"Oh, you are *that* Anne.
My neighbor still talks about you,
how you helped him
get through that terrible time."

My First Death

This spring I'm nineteen, a student nurse working
the night shift, me with twenty-six patients.
Mr. Burnett, an old farmer, almost well from
gall bladder surgery, rises early to sit with me
as I nod over charts. But this morning, his call light
blinks. I find him, his face oatmeal, his breath a whistle.

It's ten years before "Code Blue" or CPR,
so I call the intern, hoping he won't go back to sleep.
Gordon bursts in just as Mr. Burnett rattles
his last gasp. "Get me Epi and a long needle."
He pounds Mr. Burnett's chest while the drug
slips from my sweaty hands, rolls under the bed.
I crawl though dust, whispering, *"Please, God, please."*

Like a crazed killer, Gordon stabs for the heart,
hits a rib, the silver needle arcs before he slams
it home. Sparked by the curls on Gordon's nape
as he leans over the patient, a warm honey oozes
across my belly. Even as I curse my traitor's
body, I will my patient's heart to jump-start.
But Gordon shakes his head, and I hear sobs.

Mr. Burnett's son leans against the wall,
his face a gargoyle. I dart past him, my teeth
clattering as if I've been caught in murder.
I should have stayed, I should have put my arm
around his shoulders, but I am as green to death
as the jonquils coming up on the hospital lawn.

Sondercommando

*Sondercommando: Jewish prisoners who
worked in concentration camps.*

At a benefit for a wild bird sanctuary
people gnaw ribs to a blues band.
In chicken wire cages pelicans squawk,
hop, peck at dry dirt. One teeters on
a single leg. One circles, dragging
its broken wing. Another, a chick in its beak,
beats the yellow body flat against a rock,
and it's 1961 again. I'm nineteen,
a student nurse at Central State Hospital,
a jailer's keys hanging from my belt.
On the men's ward, psychopaths herd
schizophrenics through the showers,
shave the slack faces of catatonics.
In the dayroom a screened TV blares.
Patients stagger in orbit, rock in corners,
or argue with unheard voices while I play
gin rummy with joking psychos, soon
forgetting who has murdered, who has raped.
On Fridays patients from the chronic wards
pour into the gym. An inmate band saws
hillbilly tunes while I bump bellies
with Jesus, Napoleon, and sweaty men
who gallop or drool on my starched bib.
Other days I lead muttering women,
shuffling like Mother after her shock
treatments, to have their brains fried.
When the doctor turns on the juice,
I feel like a Jew herding loved ones
to the ovens at a death camp, holding down
a bucking arm or leg. At night, I wake
from a dream of maimed birds and wait
for a voice to order me to hand over
my keys, to join my kind in the pen.

6

Dry Drowning

He comes walking into the ER, holding
hands with a wife and a little boy.
A big guy, he's wheezing like
a pump organ in a country church.
"I'm thirty-five today. It's my asthma."
I put him on a stretcher, start inhalers,
get a page in to the ER doc, an IV going,
shoot some epinephrine, but the dumb
galoot stops breathing. Laryngiospasm.
I grab a lung man who's walking by.
He intubates, and I squeeze that ambu bag
like a pastry chef icing a wedding cake,
but the man's lungs aren't getting air,
his blood pressure rockets. Now his heart
flutters, stops. We pump his chest,
shock him—again and again—nothing
but a straight line. Thirty minutes after
he arrives we pronounce him. His wife
and kid wait in reception, expecting
him to amble out with a birthday grin
ready for songs and cake. What they get
is me and some strange doctor, our faces
wearing the news. I drive home, waiting
to draw my next breath, and the next.

Intensive Care

You were going to show
your boy how a man rides.
Instead you taught him
how to fly. Sailing
over handlebars,
did you see the sky
swirl to meet concrete,
feel your head splatter
like a melon? Now
bound in hospital white,
your muscles rev with power.
You are Evel Knievel
over Snake River Canyon
a Hell's Angel with
teeth strung like scalps
from your belt. The bed
rises in a giant wheelie.
You fly this new chopper
through nurses, needles
mummy wrappings on
a road only you can see.

Work, What It Is

When the alarm howls like a hungry
coyote, it's still night out. I stagger
from bed, slide into scrubs,
ignore coffee's acid stab
on an empty stomach, race
for a good parking spot,
clip on my ID, become Nurse Anne—
not wife, not mother, not me—
match boxes of time to stuff
that won't wait—meds, dressings,
patients to walk, those complaining
puppets—run against the clock, stop
everything for this doctor, that PA,
the sudden onset chest pain, trot
down the hall double time
trying to blank out thoughts
of last night's sulking child,
the quarrel, the sex we didn't have.
I make it past lunch, eyes drooping
over charts to office drone,
push myself back up to answer lights,
smile for the new admission
who puts me into overtime,
make myself think *Friday paycheck*,
drive home on clogged roads
head spinning with forgotten promises
pocketed on scraps of paper, leaving
the patients still waiting for juice,
a pain pill. I pull into the garage,
take a deep breath,
and brace myself for real life.

True Colors

My husband phones me from Costa Rica
in the shadow of the Arenal Volcano,
a growling monster I can hear thousands
of miles distant over crackling wire.
He describes chunks of molten rock
big as boxcars bouncing down the hillside,
a night sky lit by flames, bubbling lava rivers
and—click—he is gone, the phone dead.

At work I am thinking of him, when Mr. Gleason,
a coronary bypass patient I had just seen,
turns on the call light. I find a canyon
in his chest, an infected sternal wound
laid open by festered muscle, rotted sutures.
A wayward finger of bypassed artery
waves free; the walls sparkle, sprayed
gang-war red. Mr. Gleason's dead eyes stare.

My husband comes home to me unsinged,
but I am scarred, as if by Arenal.
I tiptoe around boiling pots, honed blades,
drive slowly in the right-hand lane.
Mr. Gleason visits my dreams to remind me
of my own pulsing lava, the hidden rainbow
palate—goldenrod fat, damson spleen,
lilac intestine—and the price of opening
this thin skin sack to my own scalding beauty.

On a Roll

I've mislaid a lot of stuff lately—
a button from my new coat,
a left contact lens, my favorite pen.
Now I almost lose my husband.
He comes to me as I sleep
in a halo of bathroom light.

He dances a jig by the bed,
his voice a faint metallic whistle.
I'm a nurse, adept in CPR, certified
in advanced cardiac life support,
so I know how easy it is to die.
I'm on my feet, ready to stop
that domino cascade—
the breath, the heart, then the brain.
I hug him a la Heimlich again, again.
Still the shrill noon siren, not breath,
and he begins the float away to join
patients who've died despite my skill.
I shove him facedown over a chair back
jerk my fists into his gut hard enough
to massage his backbone. A cough drop,
sucked down with a snore, flies
into a corner. My husband lies down
already asleep, a burped baby,
while I tremble beside him, thinking
how, like the pale blue contact lens
that swirled down the drain,
he could have been lost to me forever.

Slow Night in the ER

"We've got a man with gas gangrene."
I look up from my crossword puzzle,
raise an eyebrow. Gas gangrene?
It's a couple of hick ambulance drivers
who've seen too many old movies.
But one of them is carrying a big carton
marked "O Positive," so I pay attention.
They drag in a stretcher, blood
dripping off the sides. "He was working
under a truck, and the jack slipped.
Wheel rim caught his belly."

The patient, a black man, mid-thirties,
clutches at the sheet with callused hands
when I tug it down to see something
more personal than his pecker; ropy blue
intestines studded with brassy fat spill
onto the gurney. By then I'm on the horn,
calling for orders: stuff the guts back in,
cover the yawning wound with saline-
soaked towels, pump in more blood.

I can't do it. My hands won't work.
I stand outside the curtain, shaking
till his soft voice comes at me. "Miss?
Are you there?" I glove up, put on
a big smile, walk through those drapes
like a movie star on Oscar Night,
"We're going fix you up as good as new."
I keep up the stupid grin, lifting the dead
weight of hot guts, feeding them back
into his belly's maw. "How's the pain?"
I ask. "Just a little." He points to a tiny nick
on an eyelid. I think maybe there is a God
until a week later kidney failure kills him.

Widowmaker

Seven a.m. on the post-op heart unit
morning report drones. I doodle through
all the patients but mine—Mr. Johnson
for discharge, Mr. Elton for tests,
a post-op triple bypass—gut hanging
like an old hammock, pack-a-day smoker.
Lucky wife, luckier still the guy,
his widowmaker caught before it axed him.

My buddies and I do all the right stuff,
eat our veggies, exercise. Today we hike
the Smokies on a bright leaf carpet.
Doug and I plunge ahead until he stops—
"I hear something." A loud crack shakes
the tree canopy. Overhead a hickory tilts,
snaps, raining leaves like golden eyes,
bowing to take us in its deadly arms.

Doug's wife, Janet, and I once shared a toke
for old times. As I drove home that night,
an hour passed to the first stop sign. Now
time flashes as I run from yellow death.
The forest floor thuds. I'm still standing,
but Doug lies facedown under branches.
Another moment freezes before he climbs free.
"That was almost a widowmaker," he says.

We clamor over rocks to cascading falls,
but I can't stop shaking, seeing myself
smashed, just as earlier that week I jumped
from the path of a cell-talking soccer mom
gunning her rhino SUV, inches saving me.
All weekend, we chant "widowmaker,"
a magic charm, but any nurse knows
that the tiger death is always stalking.

Modern Nursing

I work in a hospital where we speak the obscure
English dialect called Cardiology—beta blockers,
Wenckebach, Tombstone Tees. My patients wear
electronic stickers on their chests, mapping
the mysteries of their hearts while I concoct
chemical cocktails to synchronize the wavy lines.
Certified in defibrillation, cardiac conversion,
I program pumps, Doppler silent pulses,
dispense drugs from a computerized bank,
my nimble hands always cool, quick, efficient.
One day I see a film: in a Russian hospital
the nurses' station is only a portrait of Lenin
over a card table. The narrator says nurses
don't keep charts, since patients cannot sue,
says medicines and equipment are scarce.
I wonder what they can possibly do for the sick.

On vacation in Scotland I beg at the bar for ice
when my friend Sandra vomits for two days
till her kidneys fail. I ride with her to the hospital.
The ambulance driver says, "You probably want
to pay. Americans always do." The nurses ask
only her name, age, my phone number.
One room holds two rows of iron bedsteads,
a bad joke from a World War II movie. Sandra,
sicker than the rest, lies behind a screen at the end.
Beside her bed stands only an iron IV pole.
I grab a plastic chair from the pile by the door,
to sit, useless, as the nurses flutter over her
like white butterflies. The next day I find Sandra
sitting up in bed, smiling. As Mr. Pillow,
the head nurse, informs me of improved vital
signs, increased urine output, he strokes her arm.
When I go home to my job, I let my hands
linger on a shoulder, warm a wrist, knowing
now that it all comes down to this, the touch.

A History of Nursing

Immune to flies and smell
I cruise back wards, listing
casualties with a practiced eye.
Bodies of men glisten with
iced sweat. Yet, hearing
my long skirts rustle between
cots, they move hands to cover
soft hearts of sex, leave
open the grin of wounds.
In front wards the sun
blinds me, glinting off
yellow mums and waxed
floors. Neatly bandaged men
greet me with smiles pinned on
like medals. Sitting among
straight bed rows, I speak
of the future of nursing—
my womanly art, the fight
against sepsis. As I talk
a red stain creeps under
the locked door and soaks the hem
of my immaculate white dress.

White

At first white means bride dolls, the snow
that falls once or twice each winter.
Then it becomes the lacy dress
I wear in the baptismal pool,
cotton bras and tampons, the shoes
called white bucks my boyfriend scuffs
under my grandmother's scrutiny.

The spring I'm fifteen, Grandmother
takes me to a place where white burns.
Mother lies under spotless sheets.
Her head flops, black hair gleams
with silver. Her eyes, the sclera shining
and wet, slide over me, never pausing.
Drugs and shock white-out memory.

Almost a woman, I leave her for a starched
uniform in a world that worships white.
I learn to strap metal onto foreheads,
to ignore the bovine bleat of patients,
biting on rubber, to hold down jerking
legs and arms. As if a white-hot current
could erase a dead father, her drunken husband.

Mother's Bible shows an old God
wearing a sparkling beard, a milky robe,
but my heaven becomes the drifting snow
I ski on Colorado slopes under peaks
like hands folded in prayer. I choose
this aching white over the fluffy clouds
through which Mother, clawing, fell.

Two

.

Mother & Daddy in Sepia

Like his Rebel grandfather, he stands
brass buttoned on the roof
of Georgia Military College.
In his hands a saxophone gleams
dully in the after "Taps" dusk.
He points the wide mouth at a flush
of lights icing the nearby College
for Women. One yellow pane hides
a girl so close that Sweet William
is her perfume, and the pulse of her
throat is just beyond his touch.
He pushes out with the horn, a long
honeyed sound. In her room, the girl
sits writing in her small neat hand.
Her eyes mirror the desk lamp
as she dreams of the dean's list
and Sunday's parlor visit. Again,
she sees his muscles moving beneath
sharp creases as he sits the hard chair.
The blaze of his smile and his crackling
black eyes touch her through woolly
uniform folds. Her breath comes short
and her writing slows. She leans
ruddy curls against a white arm,
caught in a gilt frame of sound.

The House on Bolton Road

I drive past it on the way to the airport.
Shabby men lounge with their cigarettes
on the front steps. The vast spread of grass
where I built small towns with acorns
in the roots of an absent fir tree has shrunk
to a weedy strip only yards from the street.
Instead of a rabbit warren rooming house,
I see the brick fortress, my grandmother
Annie's house, her gift from a mail-order groom,
a dirt farmer turned insurance salesman.

I want to turn in the driveway, tell the guys,
"I used to live here. Can I come in and look around?"
I would walk up those steps, past the screen porch
where Annie taught me how to crochet doilies,
into the living room, chairs circled like wagons
around a wood stove, down the long hall,
make a left turn to the kitchen where a heart attack
took my grandfather, where I sat after school
in first grade listening to Stella Dallas,
watching Annie push her weight into the handle
of a grinder, making meat loaf for supper
while my parents worked downtown.

My big sister and I slept across from the kitchen,
in the room where Annie's parents had died,
the refuge my sister shoved me from when
she heard noises in the night. Again, I tiptoe
down the haunted hall past Annie's snoring,
past Reggie Sue, the boarder, to the front room
to wake our parents. I would find them there,
still beautiful, in their thirties with jet hair,
wrapped in each other's arms, innocent as me
at six of the time when whisky would drive
a stake through the heart of their marriage
and Daddy would sit among men like those
on the steps, trying to warm himself in the sun.

My Father's War

If General George was father of
our country, my father was big chief
on the home front. The Army looked
past his straight back as they
listened to his murmuring heart.
When they wouldn't let him join
their war, he went down to the muddy
Chattahoochee and sat quietly,
awaiting that subtle pull on the line.

One day each week he spent hoeing
his yard full of corn, tinting his skin
with red clay and sun. At night
my father crept on moccasined feet,
his obsidian eyes gleaming as he
searched the house for firewater.
He fought his way through jobs
like land mines, each one growing
more treacherous. Sometimes he lay
in the mud for days, his fatigues
decorated with permanent stains.

My uncle, the colonel, cried
when my father's body declared
war on itself. But my father sat
on the riverbank and smiled,
ignoring the rocket burst of cancer
in his head. The water soaked into
his feet, made lakes of his lungs.
Dreaming of fast ponies and scalps,
he slid under the swift current.

The Birthmark

A toddler, I stand on the frontseat,
my arm around Daddy's neck as he drives,
studying that small brown island on my ribs.
It hovers over training pants pulled high
on a round belly while his voice rumbles
yarns about Scottish ancestors, Cherokee wives,
braves lurking in the woods behind our house.

I'm six when Daddy takes me to squat
on a riverbank with cane poles. He shows me
how to thread protesting worms on a hook,
how to cast a line. We compare the sun's stain
on our arms, as brown as my birthmark, unlike
the moonscape skin Mother and my sister wear.

On my eleventh birthday Daddy gives me a basketball.
Weeks later he leaves, lost to the white man's poison.
Soon that brown spot, my bit of Indian, disappears
under a jutting breast. But when I glimpse it
in the mirror, I remember his Old Spice and
tobacco smell, and miss his sweaty arm around me,
as if we had shot hoops only moments ago.

Learning to Live with It

"Please, let me stay home." I press
both hands below my navel, squeeze
out one hot tear, but Mother's
mouth freezes in a straight line.
Wearing her office clothes—nylon
over lace, clattering sling backs—
she pushes me out ahead of her,
turns the key a final click.

Now, the hard points of my butt
aching on a wooden seat, I watch
Mrs. Burns, my seventh grade
teacher. Her face turns that
purply red. This time she aims
her ruler at Robert Reynolds.
He bounces in his seat like a ball
on a bolo bat, wearing a silly smile
that only makes her screech louder.

I slide down, legs in the aisle,
yanking out my eyelashes
by twos and threes. Each little
jerk helps me forget the spit
dried at the corners of the teacher's
mouth, her whistling ruler,
how my daddy moved out,
how, ever since, my mother's
sobs rise up through the linoleum
to shake my bed at night.

Sunday Prayer

Tomato-ripe at twelve
she sways in the oven air
of church, her dress sticking
like licked candy. Up front
the deacon's voice drones
as women beat at flies with
cardboard faces of Jesus.
River-washed sinners face
the floor. Light bounces
off bent wire curls. Bald
heads shine like ceramic.

She alone looks up
to see the song leader,
a hot-rod hero saved by
the Call. Her eyes glide up
legs skimmed with Sunday
white, brushing his secret
bulge, to arms hung from
dark half moons. She stops
at his mouth, now moist
with amens, and her lips
move in silent prayer
as his eyes meet hers.

Initiation

1. Kissing Practice

When Patricia Cox, my best friend, and I hear
Barbara Bennett is going to play spin the bottle
at her birthday party, we panic. Until now,
in the seventh grade, we only had to flounder
blindfolded with a donkey tail. Kisses meant
the dry pecks of sisters and parents. Our faces
sprouting pimples, our chests crab apple breasts,
we decide to practice—the real thing. Copying
movie smooches, we press lips together—
slightly open, softened—fitting noses sideways
in a smooth glide, tongues only a nasty rumor.

2. The Real Thing

A week before that party two ninth-grade boys
give us a ride home from a basketball game.
"This isn't the way," I say, but they stop the car
on a dark road. The boy with me in the backseat,
tall tan Jesse, takes me in his arms, while his
frontseat buddy reaches for Pat. *At least a chance
to show off,* I think when his dry lips descend,
hard on mine. As if by an offstage cue, they
shove us, Pat and me, onto our backs. Jesse
jerks down my underpants. I push at his hands,
hearing only bursts of breath from the frontseat.

A filthy secret lies between my legs, a wet pad.
In the dark my face blazes. As I swat at Jesse,
my hand brushes something alive, velvet over bone.
I jerk away. He touches the pad, recoils, too, before
pressing me down again with his steely arms.
"Wait, wait. Let's talk about this," I say, and he,
daunted by that bloody lump, stops. But, hearing
his pal's grunts, he falls on me, his hard thing jabs
against the bone over my crotch, stabbing blindly
between pubic hair and pad, bruising blue pain.

3. Ever After

Finally they let us pull our panties up, skirts down.
At home I wave to my mother who sits guard by
the black phone, lie in bed wishing for Pat's chuckle,
how talking to her will make those boys a bad dream.
The next day I see Pat in the school restroom.
"What happened?" I ask, searching her gray eyes
in the mirror, but they are flat as closed doors. She,
the sharer of every secret, says, "Nothing," and turns
her back to me. Even as whispers swirl, staining
our names, I lose her forever, my best friend.

My Mentor

Mr. Trimble, I think of you often,
with the half-sized fingers dangling
from your left sleeve as you wrote on
the chalkboard with your normal right hand.
The thick glasses that slid down your nose,
the receding hairline. But mostly
I remember how you were the only person
who saw more than a poor girl at a rural school,
how you alone protested when I announced
nursing school. "Such a waste," you said.
Only you mourned when I gave my life
to a man, to children, to a boring job.
With each small victory—an aced exam,
a promotion, a publication—I whisper,
"See what I have done, Mr. Trimble."
Now forty years later, I think of you
and wonder if you, too, were forced
to compromise. I want to find you and ask,
"Mr. Trimble, is this enough?"

Body Sculpting

I raise hand weights and watch my reflection,
muscles bunching in brown shoulders, arms
drawing controlled arcs. I stand among other
lean women intent on defining sinewy curves
that once only men dared to claim, men
like my father, his shoulders strong enough
to raise me overhead. "Feel this," he would flex
biceps, tan skin over stone. "Promise me,
you'll never paint your fingernails red,
you'll always be my little buddy."

As if that could have kept him from the hooch
he loved more than me. Rain-clear sweat streams
down my face, not the tannic booze my bad
father swallowed. But his same hunger drives me
to pump out reps, willing fibers to tear and burn.
Ignoring my mother's dark curls and sad eyes,
I stare at thighs, carved like his, as if I could
bring him back, or even be him, the good father.

Two Girls Named Alice

Two friends of twenty years, as at home
in New York as Atlanta, we cab down
to the Village for a matinee. Mrs. Klein
used her own children to practice
new analytic theory: the son walks
off a cliff; the daughter, also an analyst,
vows revenge on her mother for forcing
sex, like worms, down her young throat.

Over cappuccino we rehash the play.
Suddenly my friend reveals a child
whose parents, drifting on clouds
of politics and porn, forgot her. At ten,
her father eyed her new breasts
until she backed away, stumbling into
a sinkhole. She shows me the memory
like black dirt still under her nails.

I tell her: my mother caged me
with a Baptist will against sniffing boys.
Yet at sixteen, I perched on her bed,
as she crooned about her first sex
since my father. Her legs danced against
the sheets as she asked, "Do a lot of
orgasms mean I'll get pregnant?"

She asked me, a girl who only knew
poking knees and hot breath in my ear.
I stared at the dark nest bared by
her hiked-up gown, the white belly rising
above it, and dreamed of a place safe
from that voice, oozing from her red lips.
I wanted, like my friend, to fall deep
into the ground, to huddle with other
children, fleeing parents such as ours.

Miss Edna Faye Stone

Somebody told me that you were dead,
but it's not true. You live forever
in the stone Home Ec building, where
you bully Tucker High girls into
sewing useless aprons, baking gummy pies.
You taught my class Sex Ed, passing
around a Kotex to watch us cringe,
as if we were touching a frog
or maybe a boy's creepy thing.
You talked about tubes and ovaries
cycles and shed linings, not fat,
sloppy tongues pushing past our teeth,
blind hands crawling under our clothes
or the stab of a boy's dick against
a girl's nylon underwear.
You sat, your billows of arm flesh
quivering, thundercloud thighs
slammed shut over a petrified hymen,
pointing at diagrams that had
nothing to do with me and your
so cute nephew, Chipper, or the bottle
of Jergens in the glove compartment
of his shiny black convertible,
the better to grease his way into me.
That night I smiled at myself
with puffy lips in the bathroom
mirror and thought of you, Edna Faye,
and that fleshy mole at the corner
of your mouth, the three bristles
that quiver when you grin.

Triangulation

Triangulation: The use of two known
coordinates to determine the location of a third.

On my sixth birthday, I stand by a trash fire
clutching the bride doll in white lace
Santa brought me the day before.
We've lost our home on Gladstone Road
in Atlanta because of Daddy's drinking.
Mother has to find a job when we move
three miles to live with Grandmother Annie,
but I only think of my doll and my new
cowgirl outfit with the fake leather fringe.
Wherever we live, I sleep, curled up
in the maple bed beside my big sister.

On my fifty-sixth birthday, snow glitters
as I snooze on a futon in Colorado, snug
in my daughter's house, while three miles
away in the foothills a six-year-old
beauty queen dies, a cord around her neck,
her head bashed, her underwear bloodied.

On my next birthday, I sleep at home,
three miles from Gladstone Road,
three miles from Annie's brick fortress,
and three miles from where the dead girl's
parents now live. I wake, still pulsing
from a dream of sex with a man as powerful
as Daddy, to think of that child, her TV image—
painted face and dyed hair, dancing
in a cowboy hat and fringed skirt—
frozen at the age of flat-chested dreams.
I know now, despite Daddy's drunk driving,
bouncing off mailboxes, Mother's weeping,
my sister's shrieks, I had always been safe.

A Cake to Celebrate

Today is Grandmother's birthday. Born over
a century ago, she's been dead a dozen years,
but I can still see her knotted hands pulling
greens in the garden, shelling peas,
crocheting, never resting. I write poems,
but will anyone in the next century
remember the lilt of my words as I relish
the memory of one bite of her cake,
the feathery yellow layers held together
with tart lemon curd, wearing a gossamer
white coat and a snowstorm of fresh coconut?

She tried to teach me. Set out eggs and butter
the night before. Use a hammer to crack open
the hairy coconut head into jagged chunks.
Grate the meat into fine wet flakes, beat six eggs,
each for two minutes, whip the batter on high
to liquid gold, clap pans on the table to pop bubbles
before interment in a hot oven. Tiptoe around
the kitchen as if in church while you boil icing
until it spins a silk thread that balls in water.
I do each step, but my cakes never come out
like hers, fluffy and moist, the taste of eternity.

My teenage years I lived with Grandmother
in the big yellow farmhouse while Mother,
her sorrow fried by electroshocks, wept,
jabbered, and scratched me like a cornered cat
when I took my turn sitting suicide watch.
"Not my child, you won't," Grandmother told
doctors to Mother's lobotomy. She dressed me,
the orphan of a drunk father, a crazy mother,
in handmade finery. Her sure touch fitting
a dress to my body, like the frosting
that held together her cakes, kept me from
flying to pieces. While Mother healed,
I became yet another cake in her oven.

A String of Beads

For Annie, my grandmother

Hanging from a tram strap in Prague, I look down
on a seated woman. Amber beads, clear as honey,
lie on fine white skin and floral lawn drapes
her lap. I stare at her wide-brimmed straw hat,
a hat like you wore, Annie, in my favorite picture.
The brim's shadow veils your face, your chin
framed by a feather boa. I rock on my heels,
remember other trolley rides, my hand in yours.
You could have taught me more than how to crochet,
how to play a winning game of Chinese checkers.
You survived two wars, a dead baby, a husband
gasping and blue by the kitchen stove,
your life forced like paper whites in January.
This Czech woman lived the Velvet Revolution.
Her life evolves as Prague emerges with barnacles
of new growth on ancient houses adorned with
statuary like wedding cakes. The tram window
flashes on street musicians, Marlboro signs.
A careful woman, she looks straight ahead, safely
contained by beads, a proper summer dress,
and the shade of her hat barely covers her smile.
If only I could ask her secret, your secret,
Annie, of how to live in a world flying apart.

To Mother,
On Your Eighty-third Birthday

In an old newspaper clipping you dance in a chorus line,
a dozen girls in a fashion show. It was 1931, the Depression,
yet you sport the latest style—an open coat skimming
a slim dress. Sixteen, dark curls shining, your smile
earns you the title, "prettiest girl in Atlanta." Soon you
would go off to Milledgeville, to the Georgia State College
for Women, but the following year your "sadness" would
keep you home, beginning a downward spin. Stop here.

I want to rewrite your future, to start again at the time when
you counted, like pearls on a silk string, how many dates
you could squeeze into a weekend. My new film
would show you, nineteen again, at the altar beside one of
the other men who courted you, not my father, the darkly
handsome Donald, his eyes burning into you like lava.
This husband would be sober, balding, too busy at the office
to notice the dresses you bought for me and my sister,
the sweet, obedient girls of this other father, a man who
would thank God every day for his good luck in having you.

See, I've torn up the old script, the one that shows Donald,
slipping from your arms toward a whisky bottle, that shows you,
after the divorce, taking the job you would hate, where smarter
than the rest, you trained men for promotion over you. I would
edit out the part where after work you scrub clothes in a bathtub,
cry in your lonely bed, blaming yourself for Donald's gutter slide.
Instead of the pills and barbiturates you swilled to still your frantic
hand-wringing, instead of the shock treatments, the threatened
lobotomy, you would be the grace note at dinner parties,
entertaining friends with accounts of your vacations in Europe.

The old reel shows you marrying again, to a mountain man
disguised in city clothes, a man who dragged you away from
shopping and concerts, who had you can beans from his garden,
cook for his relatives, who slapped you around when the sex stopped.
I wouldn't have to carry your whispered messages to Donald.
In my new version, you would spend afternoons reading
to a book club, wearing a new hat, a watermelon-red dress,
your pretty feet set off by sling backs. Other days your fingers
would fly over the keys of the black Royal, writing stories and poems.

Instead of swallowing a bottle of pills at sixty when I told you
Donald was dying of cancer, you would take your writing
to a beach house in winter, to a lake house in summer where
your grandchildren would visit, and I wouldn't be standing
on dead grass over your grave on a hill in North Carolina, away
from everything you loved. No. Your family would celebrate you
on this special day. You would be lovely with your crown
of thick white curls, as we come bearing gifts for the woman
who wants for nothing—handmade cards from the children,
a diamond bracelet from your doting husband—and you would
smile radiantly, like that girl in the browning newsprint.

Suicide Club

For Jalaine

You and I were flat-chested little brats,
too young for secret societies, hardly
speaking to each other on the school bus,
when my sister, at fourteen, started her own
select club. Our country school had no
sororities, just Future Farmers and Bible
Study Club, so she called it Eta Pi.

New members painted their pointy little
knockers with fingernail polish, went
to school without their underpants.
I told on my sister one night at dinner
after she ratted on me for playing
doctor. I didn't bother to tell you,
Jalaine, about how I got her grounded.
You were a kid, a whole year younger.

But listen, Jalaine, I'm telling you now.
We share more than faded yearbooks
as members of our own nasty girls' club,
too new for rules or secret handshakes.
Enrollment is automatic, sort of like
the gray hair we rinse away, but not so
easy to hide, what with the red clots
of sleepers my mother gulped, the oozing
bullet holes your folks wore to bed.

Like my sister's once-lacquered tits,
we both wear a scarlet "S" branded
on our hearts. At our meetings,
when we bother, we knock back yet
another martini, pretend we can forget
how it all got started, this bonding
of women whose parents reach out
from the grave to club them with guilt.

The Keeper

My parents lie in the dusty cage
of memory like once brilliant
jungle snakes. An occasional
sequin-bright scale shines
through yellowed skin. Too many
years of captivity, a steady
diet of rats, have bloated
their slender forms. All that is
left of the Belle is an elegantly
tapered tail. The sparkle of wit
can only be imagined in the slow
nodding of the male's ponderous head.

But I have saved a ragged
brochure. Here. They are shown
on a tree limb, in full color,
along with a description of
their feeding and mating habits.
There are fewer requests to see
them of late, though the rustle
of their coils still commands
a chill, and venom can be seen
dripping from bared fangs. I
continue to open the museum
door each morning at nine.

Letter to a Dead Father

I got out the easy way when Mother left you.
I was eleven, but my sister, sixteen, eloped
to escape clanking bottles between sofa cushions,
your nightly gorilla rampages, only to live with
another kind of brute. Without your slurred curses,
random backhands, and Mother's weeping
I slept alone, wrapped in velvet silence.

For a long time it was enough. Then I began
to forget your monster rages and remembered
your tremulous tenor crooning love songs,
you, bending Mother over in movie kisses—
"The most beautiful woman in the world"—
pulling quarters from my ears, my pal,
teaching me to plant corn and bait a hook.

Mother warned me against your kind,
while she still mourned you, her Valentino,
and her dreams—a house with white columns,
a canopied bed, candlelit dancing. Yet she wed
a man dull as the earth he farmed. When I
told her cancer grew in your lungs like kudzu,
she wore a lacy gown to swallow all her pills.

Now I have what Mother wished for me, Daddy,
the opposite of you. This man, blonde to our
Cherokee dark, shines, gold flakes in sand,
weighs each word for truth. Even after forty years
this Marine is as likely to speak Urdu as utter
sweet lies and braces himself against the gale
of my kisses. His blue eyes still melt my bones.

But I yearn for one last waltz around the kitchen,
standing atop your feet, the brush of your fingers
against my cheek as if my skin were rose petals.

Three

Burial

In 1968 Barbara Jane Mackle, an Emory coed, was kidnapped
and buried for three days before her rescue.

My name is Beautiful Barbara
and I live in a box. Once
I lived outside, but I
couldn't get off my leash.

Like sheep to the slaughter,
like Jews to the ovens,
I leave my mother's thin arms,
a Southern girl chloroformed.
Better to live in the ground than sin.

My trousseau is red flannel,
a sweater for warmth. "The light
is here, food there, an alarm button
in case anything goes wrong."
Now I lay me down to sleep.

I hear screws twist. Habits,
children fall like dirt
onto the lid of my coffin.
Stupid, I lie here and dream
of stubby fields, running, running.

The wood is hard against my bones,
cold needles my feet. I suck
at drafts and fumble for the button.
The alarm breaks off in my hand.
Dear God, my name is Beautiful Barbara
and I live in a box.

The Exhibitionist

We are carnival freaks
you and I. My priapism
hides behind soft lips
a phantom limb engorged
with secret dreams. There
you stand, knowing somehow
I must drive this way.
I see you. Your jet of come
glitters in the sun like
broken glass, your eyes
rivet mine. Yes, I am
your sister, turned inside
out, dark caves glistening.
So often you visit my nights
with your soft look
your one-eyed monster.

Eating

is the only bodily function
we can do in polite company,
not tooth or nose picking,
hawking up globs, scratching
butts, balls, labia, inspecting
the contents of any body crevice
gleaned with a fingernail.
But there are rules: eating must
be done discretely, mouth closed,
no talking. Remember, farting
is not allowed, even among friends.
The wine, the coffee, the tasty
chewables we swallow must soon
make a private splash in the toilet,
as secret as the rut-humping sex
we do with others—or alone—
behind closed doors. So all that's
left is to sit up straight, one hand
in my lap, trying not to cram in the
good stuff, like the animal I am.

When in Paris

How long since that man tailed me through a parking lot,
his gaze fixed on my legs? I thought of him last week
when sex sparked in a colleague's eyes, fed by
my breasts taut against fabric. I had almost forgotten
the power that lights men's eyes. In America, a woman
over fifty, like a cozy couch, escapes notice.

Oh, whistles ring from passing cars, and drivers'
hormones throb with rap's bass thump, until they see
my face, their mother's face. Still, friends' husbands
squeeze me too tight, like a taste of Swiss chocolate.
Older men look twice, for a moment forgetting wives
and progeny, silver-backed apes near their end.

But in Paris, young men's eyes caress, their smiles glide
over me like silk. My hostess tells me, "Here in France
we have a tradition: a woman teaches a friend's son
about love." Is that why she leaves me alone with her
towering child? In morning sun his stubble gleams black,
the whites of his eyes shine blue as breast milk. Fine hairs
on his hands catch light, and he turns his gaze on me.

Mein Liebes Deutschland

I wear chunky rubber-soled shoes, a pea-green coat
I bought at the Kaufhaus, a scarf twisted around
my neck like the locals. Give me credit. Not many
Americans try your punishing Prussian vocals.
I chew on your taffy words, cough up strings
of the stuff with Bach or ach, while goo blocks
my sinuses. I've learned to pretzel sentences till verbs
kiss nouns at the back door and spit consonants
like tacks until they blister the tip of my tongue,
yet my accent stays as flat as Hamburg's horizon.
Still you spurn me with a sideways glance
and answer my questions in perfect English.
When we meet over glasses of beer, you tempt me
with glimpses of pale Nordic flesh. Yet little do
you know how I restrain myself from popping
you one, you, a strutting peacock, sneering
at my stories' rose-colored endings. I ask myself,
too, *Why don't I stay where I belong?*
Your garbled verbiage was going to be my ticket
to the big picture, but now I'm hooked on the misery,
whipping myself nightly with knotted cords of verbs,
bleeding in a hair shirt of nouns' uncertain gender.
When we dance, you press me to your chest, Mein
Liebes, and whisper, *"Aggressive American woman."*

Husband Shaving

Bouncing up the stairs
I imagine a hard curve
of hip. He stands naked
a jet of lather on his palm.
Paths of pink satin gleam
cut through foam. Biceps bunch
as he feels for strays.
I think how my circling hands
will sift curls on his chest,
cradle soft cups of seed,
my hardening nipples sweep
his smooth back. I know
he will turn, his mouth
will search me, leave trails
of white. Before I reach
the bathroom door, my legs
dissolve, soap in water.

"Self Portrait" At the Whitney Biennial

After a photograph by Catherine Opie

A woman wears a black leather hood so tight
that it shrinks her brain, flattens her face.
Her chin juts over squared shoulders, hands
rest on hips, her lower half cut off by frame.
Steel bolts pierce her long brown nipples.
She stares at me through slits in the hood
as if she is ignoring the hypodermic needles
threaded through the skin of her outer arms
at precise intervals like tin soldiers marching,
their razor tips pressing out ruby drops.

I imagine her: barely a woman, she kneels
before an altar, offering the white nape,
her shaved head, as Chinese girls hold out
their feet to be bound. She promises to love
and obey, accepting, as the laces tighten,
a man's promise to protect. He keeps her safe,
her skull squeezed to fit house and babies,
safe from demons of choice, unruly desire.

Behind the hood, her cheeks bunch in a smile.
She proudly wears the medals earned by decades
with one man. Wired for pleasure, she is
chained by years of regular orgasms gotten
the way she likes best, to babies pushed out
below her frame, the gilt house her man has built.
If she could speak, I would ask her:
How has my long marriage marked me?
Do my wounds glisten like yours?

Becoming Myself

A woman on *Cybil*, a sitcom, explains why she looks so young:
"The plastic surgeon has cut away enough loose skin to make a small fat person."

When I was twenty-five I stared at skin
sagging over the eyes of another nurse,
more than twice my age, and vowed
I'd never allow anything so sloppy
happen to me. I sucked in my gut,
ran a rat maze of daily miles, banked
orgasms against the day when men would
turn away in the neverland of menopause.

So who is that woman in the latest
family photo? Her lids droop worse
than those of my early colleague.
The nose, the hair are mine, yet a sneaky
side view reveals an accordion neck
never seen in the makeup mirror.
I glimpse Age creeping around the corner
on rubber-soled shoes, hoping to rob
this woman of all she holds dear.

But I have a surprise for him.
I don't need old tricks of tight skin.
My power comes from a head crammed
with knowing, a body proud of its years.
I smile when a young colleague,
her skin like wedding china,
stares at my earned wrinkles.
I can almost hear her silent oath.

My Husband Retires

I've counted down the years on my fingers,
now the day I've dreaded has come—
your liberty, my chaos. Thick blonde hair
and a flat belly prove you too young,
yet you pocket the pension, a lump sum
radioactive with possibilities.
All I have to do is nod: you would drag me
to dusty Alabama, a farm by a pond
of jumping bass, a log cabin in Montana,
windows blinking at the Beartooth Range,
a beach house on the tenth hole of nowhere.
"Where do you want to go?" I say.
"If you knew me, you wouldn't have to ask."
With money that must last forever,
we fly to Ireland. A week in the car,
our eyes numbed by rocky beauty,
talk dwindles to a thin line of spittle.
In a pub a man says he never locks a door.
"I love it here," you say, raising your pint
to the farmer in manure-smeared boots.

Later we stand in a forty-mile wind
one step from the edge at the Cliffs of Moher.
The sea boils six hundred feet below.
The writer in me imagines the story, a mystery—
the shove to a shoulder, the waiting rocks—
but I wrap my arms around your solid waist
as we look out toward America. I know
now where you would live out our years—
not in Montana or Alabama—but the fifties
where housewives vacuum in heels, men
doff fedoras, and I am safe, here in the nineties.

Exoskeletons

Admiring the order of its plated shell, I watch a turtle's
plodding progress through the backyard impatiens bed.
Intent on gaining a spot of moist shade, the turtle
inches along, ignoring nearby hammering. In the garage
my husband clears out detritus of twenty years—
scattered hammers and screws, bits of board, empty boxes.

He's been at it for days now, only stopping for a beer,
the odd meal. Garbage cans overflow. Shelves appear,
tailored for paint cans, electrical gear, and his father's
old gizmos. Giveaways pile up where his car used to park.
At midnight I peek out to tell him good-night,
but, as if meeting a deadline, he stays up to sort rusty nails.

I rise early to pounding. A new rack for folding chairs
juts overhead. Once-jumbled tools, now ordered
like a tray of surgical instruments, lie in pristine rows.
Until months ago he wore a captain's stripes, commanding
an airborne ship. He began as an ace in an orange jumpsuit,
skimming the desert floor at five hundred miles an hour,
immortal under the dome of an attack bomber.

His bride, I stood beside a runway watching him fly
touch-and-go landings, my body vibrating from engine noise,
bathed in hot exhaust, knowing that night I would sleep
with a jock Marine. Thirty-five years later, he salutes
the ground crew on his last flight and walks away forever
from his hero's aura. Now he structures a new life,
making his house as orderly as that turtle's neat shell.

An Irish Stroll

"What would you like to do?" he asks.
"A long stroll on the Burren," I say.
And so I get my way; he trudges,
back rounded. "Pretend you're playing golf,"
I tell him. I know he hates walking
not done on fairways. Once a Marine,
any exercise must have purpose.
Shoulders of silver stone rise over Europe's
western arm. From crevices where oceans
once flowed, alpine blooms and tropical
flora spring. Genetians wink brilliant
blue eyes, purple orchids on two-inch stems
beg to be picked. I dare to break stride,
to look a sunny primrose in the eye, touch
a tiny velvet fern. He checks his watch,
taps his toe. "We've walked forty minutes."
"Just a little farther," I say, "around that bend."
"We'll walk till you can't take another step."
Smiling, I take the lead and pick up the pace.
I'd almost forgotten how much he loves me.

Thirty-six Years

For Larry

52

We stood at the altar so long ago,
as if at Mount Katahdin in Maine,
starting at the wrong end
of the Appalachian Trail, too young
to worry about hunger or bears,
tipped groundward by backpacks
loaded with useless gear.
We have slogged over boulders,
creek beds, thankless mountains,
looking only at our trudging feet,
to break open before an occasional vista
with the world opened up at our boots.
Sometimes you take the lead,
other times I do—until we can hardly
remember anything but this trail.
Losing sight of each other for hours,
one of us, breathless, always catches up,
happy the sight of a familiar shape means
we are not lost, at least from each other.
But now we are on the downhill slope,
almost to the trailhead at Springer Mountain
where we will burst free in a meadow
leading to hot showers and real beds.
The sunlight through trees catches
on your blonde hair, and suddenly
I know I would choose what I chose
so long ago, this life we trek together.

The Woman My Husband Should Have Married

I know exactly what she looks like: big, perky
breasts, tight, little waist and long blonde hair.
This woman likes to cook. Every night she
serves him a feast of fresh vegetables, fried
chicken or steak, minus the lectures about arteries
slamming shut. Her idea of fun is watching him
ride his tractor around their farm in south
Georgia where she sews and makes preserves
when not entertaining his relatives. She knows
all the rules of baseball and football, likes to
watch golf on TV with him on Sunday afternoons.

He cannot hurt her feelings. His sexist jokes
make her laugh until tears run. She squeezes
a dollar until it stretches like rubber, never
runs up the credit cards, not her. She dresses
like a queen in last year's clothes, always
wearing the four-inch heels he loves. She won't
let him help in the kitchen and rubs his back
when the dishes are done. She hates foreplay:
she lies back, wet and ready in ten seconds flat,
unless, of course, he prefers a blow job.

Poor guy. He got me instead. A city girl,
who lives for books, art, long slow kisses,
who hates cooking and sports. Once,
when I was gone a month, friends gave him
a blow-up doll. Now, when he walks in
that door, his pink face full of hope,
I want to be her, Marilyn Monroe in an apron,
waiting for the details of his golf game.
Instead I quietly leave him with his TV
and newspaper so he can at least pretend.

Four

The Hymn Singer

He is always waiting
at the edge of my dreams.
Metered footfalls muffle his
soft crooning—*Are you washed
in the blood?* He blesses my sleep
with the oil of his coming.
I wake as he raises the knife.

Now the ghost made flesh—
redheaded, fifteen—descends
to earth, to my little girl
in her second-grade beauty.
*Praise Him all ye little
children* is his lullaby
as he takes her in his arms.

The police bring him, charmed
with bracelets, a Bible jutting
from his pocket. Now she knows
as I know the burning print
of his face. He is humming
*Standing on the promises
of God.* Always humming.

A Girl's Father

"Daddy, stand up straight!" She pushes
at his rounded shoulders. A daughter
her body as erect as a loblolly pine
does not see that he is weighed down
like an African man under a yoke,
carrying buckets of water for miles
to keep his bloated children alive.
She does not yet know the forces that bend
people like trees under a wet spring snow.

Her father, a Marine, trained to survive
off snakes and rainwater, to shoot out
the heart on a man target, to drop bombs
on sleeping villages, wages unseen
battles. His body pumps hormones
designed for cracking small bones
with his fists, for bathing in the stink
of sweat and blood, for fucking
quickly and cruelly, faceless women.

The open road sings a siren's song:
travel light, fast, alone. The father
pretends not to hear. The daughter sees
only the shape he has taken out of love—
a trim, middle-aged man, muscles heavy,
who sighs as he mails out checks,
trudges off to a job wearing pants
now shiny in the seat, whose eyes
moisten when he holds a new baby.
He hangs up his male heart like a coat
worn only on special occasions,
now too tight across the shoulders,
and stares into a distance she cannot see.

How Does Your Garden Grow?

You grow in little jerks
my time-lapsed flower.
I watch a blue vein
begin sly swelling
under one nipple, your legs
turn to knobby stems.
Feet that once fit
into my hand lengthen
like feeder roots.
Your stalk of waist
stretches and narrows
and three dark hairs
sprout under an arm.
Coquette, you peer through
petals barely parted.

New Age Pusher

*May 1996: Rob Hall, a mountain guide, died on
Mount Everest rather than abandon a climber.*

Rob Hall had some nerve, burrowing down in a snow hole,
sucking tanks dry of oxygen to die with a tourist from Seattle.
He gave himself like a lover to the blizzard, radioed
his pregnant wife, telling her not to worry while his hands
and face became crystal. Like him, you, my daughter,
measure your goals in thousand-foot increments
of Arctic tundra, racing your bike above the Colorado tree
line over skittering gravel trails hikers can barely climb.

Your friend tells me how, at eleven thousand feet,
you skidded off a cliff, but had the luck to land on a ledge.
You shrug at India ink scars mapping your muscled legs.
"I need to be afraid," you say. I remember catgut knit
into your black brows, an arm sagging over splintered bone,
and later, inky pupils crowding out blue as you flew on dope.
And stupid me, after you had crouched, weeks alone
driving out the demon, I thought quitting drugs had saved you.

Now ten years later the devil returns, singing Rob Hall's
thin tune. While new climbers step over his iced corpse,
you shoot up danger like crystal meth, jamming the pedals
over bald peaks. I look away from hand-sized scabs, picturing
your once baby-pink skin, as you, too, tell me not to worry.
I can only bruise my knees nightly that the phone never
rings with the dreaded news, that you may live past thirty.

Room Design

My daughter asks me to help arrange
her bedroom furniture. First the futon.
Lia lifts her end like a tray of glasses.
Mine just clears the floor. We set the chest
by her bed, the white pine desk under
a window, leaving the papasan chair
to jut out like a rude comment. We hang
photos in blues and greens—Lia hiking
in Bryce Canyon, mountain biking in Moab.

In 1922, Grandmother was Lia's age—thirty.
Three toddlers hung from her skirts
like baby possums when the news came:
a drunk taxi driver, her husband dead. I asked
Grandmother how she'd survived.
"I moved furniture." Her heavy oak
sideboard perches in my garage. I think
how she shoved it, the balled feet scraping
plank floors, then pushed it back again.
The grooves underfoot mocked tear tracks
on her cheeks, just as torn muscles masked sorrow.

I sit on the futon by Lia, an engineer, single
and buoyant as any cloud. I want to tell her
how two generations have given her this life,
but just as when I describe my bra-burning days,
her blue eyes would glaze. She'd sooner understand
Egyptian hieroglyphics, my past is that ancient.

Acquittal

For those wrongs I inflicted on you, my son,
I wear guilt like a belt cinched notches too tight.
From the moment in the delivery room when
I sat on your head, pushing out of my body,
to receive the saddle block, you have suffered
to have such a mother. Still a child myself,
you became my new toy, like the doll
I'd left out in the rain ten years earlier.

These are my confessions: The day of your
birth I smiled to hide the evil thought—
I don't want to be anybody's mother. I still cringe,
remembering how, when your daddy flew jets,
I swatted at you, a kitten tugging on my leg,
ignored your little boy tricks, bopped you
with a wooden spoon for tormenting your sister.
Yet you gave me kisses, told me you would live
with me always. Your little boy voice still rings
in my ears as it once pealed across grocery aisles—
"Mommy, I love you!" I told myself not to worry,
at thirty-five you would have plenty to tell a therapist.

Now, you're nearly that age, a businessman,
when you call me at noon, your voice quivering.
"There's just one thing I can't forgive," you say.
As if in a car rolling over a precipice, time slows,
breath stops in a tide of nausea. "Tell me."
"The time Hank Aaron hit his record-breaking
home run, you didn't take me to the game."
"Oh, that's it?" At last I can draw a deep breath.

Observance

I watch you, my son, offer your baby girl
in her trailing lawn dress to the pastor,
smile when she grabs his nose and coos.
Beside you, your wife holds hands with toddler boys
who twist around her legs like tropical vines.
As you give this new child to the church,
I remember how, branded with words of Sartre,
Russell, and Maslow, I vowed to keep you free
of my childhood's curse—the fiery sermons,
a preacher's accusing finger, fear of sleep
and dying, my body forever afire for some
small sin. I threw away the hair shirt
of guilt that pushed my mother into suicide
and taught you to believe in good, not God.
Your smile for your wife, for this baby,
glows incandescent as you repeat the vows.
Your blue eyes unclouded by doubt, you never
wonder if you can raise your children to be free.

Peepee Poopoo

I hear them in the bathroom,
toddler brothers, two and three.
Water splashes, the commode
gurgles, giggles creep under
the closed door. Forbidden
words float to the kitchen where
I chop onions. "Hiney, doo doo
tee tee." One wears diapers yet.
When naked, he fingers little balls,
grins up at me. I remember at three
in the woods behind our house,
my pants off, Ben DiMayo's
around his ankles. We stared,
at each other, touched ourselves,
the burning tickle enough. Now
my grandsons wear the blueprint
in their perfect plump bodies of
muscle and sinew, of the pleasure
they will give and receive.

Getting Even

At twenty months, Jack toddles by
to lean over his little brother's downy
head as if to kiss. *So sweet,* I think,
but the baby shrieks. A red arc of teeth
marks the soft spot. Their mother snatches
up the baby, points a stiff finger at Jack.
"You are so bad!" His tears wet the pillow
as I lay the chubby boy down to sleep.
"No, ma'am, no, ma'am." Jack stings
me with his tiny arsenal of words.

You, my sister, had other ways of
punishing me. Already five when I came,
you were too tough to cry. In photos
you glare as our father holds me
to his chest. You took revenge by
vacuuming my toes, dosing me
with vanilla and pepper, reading to me—
stories about children who die in flames—
any torture that didn't leave marks.

Half a century later, stroking this little
boy's silky hair, I remember how we sisters
snuggled in our maple bed, safe together
even while our father raged and our mother
wept, the pinches, the tattling, the kicks
under the table forgotten and forgiven.
I think how someday Jack will yearn
for his brother, just as I grow hungry
for you, my sister, your voice in my ear,
your cold-creamy good-night kiss.

The Lie

A knife pushed through a bagel slips.
Blood drips from a finger, the first I've
shed in months. Changing my grandbaby's
diaper, I think of that blood. The fat halves
of her bottom meet like the seam of a peach.
"You are perfect," I tell her, just as I told
my daughter, just as my mother told me.
This child has two brothers with silky skin,
as sweet as their melted-chocolate eyes.
Yet no one feeds them that lie.
We won't tell her until whispers come
to her incredulous ears, how she will bleed,
enough in her lifetime to fill a small room,
how from the moment the first smear appears,
she will be set apart from her brothers, ruled
by the drag of bellyache, the flow she must
staunch with pads and plugs, the clothes
she checks for blotches. She will spend her life
dreading the blood, longing for the blood,
her fate written in sticky red. We won't warn her
how men, like timber wolves drawn by the scent
of her hidden core, will become her willing slaves.

Road Rage

Racing a yellow light, I honk at a woman
who pulls out then slows down.
The list on the car seat beside me
rations my minutes. I check off each item,
pen digging into paper, as if the trip
to the grocery, letters mailed, clothes
washed and folded, dishes put away
would save a life in Iraq. By dark,
the food I cook has been gulped,
a new list replaces the old. I watch Luke,
a two-year-old grandson, build a tower
of wooden blocks, knock them over,
start again. "Look at me," he commands
that night in the bathtub. He holds
two plastic cups—one yellow, one purple—
pours rivers over his head, throws cascades
into the air. "Tea party," he says, grinning.
I take the cup of murky water he offers
to toast at least one life with purpose.

Who Will Mother the Mothers?

I doze in my chair. Pots chime
in the kitchen, and I think,
Oh, it's Mother, cooking,
and sink back, forgetting
she is dead for twenty years,
and I am now the mother
of a father. I hear her:
she sings my wake-up call,
promises hot cakes and bacon
a morning of sunshine. I feel
her fingers stroke my hair
as lightly as butterflies.

Junkyard Salvage

Like stains of red wine creeping along
the threads of a linen tablecloth,
my genes hopscotch random fibers,
weaving me into a patchwork blend
of family donors. I wear my mother's
Irish eyes, a grandmother's long feet,
my father's helpless smile. Tossed
like dice from a cup, the same genes
become my sister. She wears Mother's
milky skin, along with her gift
of honing words into polished beauty.
Pieced from another quilt top, fusing
new patterns with old, my son tells
the jokes of a grandfather he never knew.
My daughter flies a bike over mountain trails
as her father once flew attack bombers.
A niece guards her box of legal drugs,
as careful in addiction as three of her grandparents.
In my arms, I study a new baby's round face,
a jigsaw puzzle of two families, and tweak
his right foot, its two fused toes matching mine.

Five

Gutshot

Captain Karen Walden is a character in
Courage Under Fire, a 1996 film.

Those early years I dreamed of this girl's fist scoring
a clean right to a jaw, of vaulting a horse from a dead run,
of shooting it out with the black hats. But even then I knew
nothing could make a hero like staying behind
with a belly full of lead, holding off the redskins
to save the women and children. Karen Walden knows.
When she drops, her stomach strafed, she orders her men
to retreat, fires her M16 at attacking Iraqis. She dies
saying her little girl's name and becomes the first
woman ever nominated for the Medal of Honor.

In a cowboy dream, the hand clutching my side holds in
guts peppered by buckshot. Blood, thick and warm,
pumps over my fingers. Now it's my chance
to hold off the Indians, to hunker down behind
my old buddy Paint while my partner heads for the hills.
As I reach for my toy six-shooter, glory fades.
I'm a woman sick with Crohn's, no hero, my family
won't cut and run, and the bullet holes in my bowel
are here to stay. I learn what Walden knew.
Dying is easy. Living hurts, and it takes a long time.

Dr. Crohn, how nice of you to lend
your name. It sounds so much better
than "Inflamed Intestinal Disease."
In your day I could have stood among
satin-skinned women and tuxedoed men,
allowing your rounded vowel to slip
like a smoke ring from my lips.
Of course, back then, cameras didn't
spy into one's most secret realms,
snap photos of colon ulcers like
postcards of shorelines for relatives.
Friends didn't ask the gritty details,
but came for short visits bearing
bouquets and chocolates. Now I gulp
slick red pills in secret and pretend
I have a malady that requires me
to wear lace and perfume,
to take long naps on chaise lounges.

74

Birthright

I inherited the McDonald constitution—
straight bones, endurance of a marathoner,
physical arrogance of a mountain lion—
from a drunk father who took falls that
would maim another man, got up and shrugged;
from a great grandmother who climbed
sixteen steps from the outhouse till she was ninety-five;
from a great-great grandfather who arrived in a Conestoga
with nine sons to carve out a new Atlanta after Sherman.

Like my wedding gift, the bracelet with an 1890 gold coin,
I lost my claim to wake up child-happy and fit,
ready to take on whatever my nurse job could demand—
hemorrhage, cardiac arrest—when a doctor delivered
the diagnosis, eclipsing the clan's protection.
My denim-blue fingers, sloshing waves of gut,
pills bitter as green persimmons, humble me
like a guilty supplicant, and I study
the family tree to wonder which of
these dead has committed this treason.

Trophy Hunters

Last week a doctor told me I'm special.
My colon, as pockmarked as a teen
with acne, is twice the normal length.
I dream of artfully draping it around
my neck like a feather boa, posing for
publicity shots, lovely in tones of rose
and lilac. But no. It lies coiled under
my belt like a snake on a cold winter day,
seen only by hunters who forage
in my dark places with flouroscopes.

Odd innards run in the family. My mother
sported one huge kidney. A horseshoe,
curled under her ribs, brought her
no protection against the depression
she deadened with drugs. I see Mother
in the mirror each morning when I gulp
my ration of reds and whites:
steroids and immune suppressors,
to calm a slack gut eating at itself.

I would gladly trade my trick intestine
for her bad luck horseshoe when
at a medical lecture I see slides:
excised colons of patients with my disease—
brittle red question marks on green towels,
piano keys of fat marching up the sides.
So I take my pills to keep the surgeon,
like some south Georgia good old boy
at a rattle snake roundup, from snatching out
my gut to show it off like a prize specimen.

Arthritis, A Lesson

I can no longer hide this secret shame.
My hands bloom into angry gloves.
Ten knuckles, one wrist sprout
bony lumps. Long nights
read like pornography:
hot swollen parts
throb, ache, tingle.
Ask me to make a fist
with these rebel fingers,
you will see how far gone I am.
I've learned to grovel at God's feet
for every small gift. At least,
the rusty nails I feel piercing
my palms don't draw blood.
He gives me that.

Moisture Seekers

An ode to Sjögren's Syndrome

"Can you swallow a Saltine dry? Are your eyes
sandstorm red?" *Don't listen to him, Anne.*
He's a doctor, not a man. He digs up
my secrets like desert fossils: crystal sharp tears,
hands curled into claws. Pulling me close,
he inspects my smooth, knobby knuckles
and hums over blue nail beds. The sound
of his gurgling belly tells me I'm already
dried up, like the four-hundred-year-old Pope
with brown parchment skin I saw in Rome.
The doctor drives nails into my coffin with a book—
it shows a man with his eyes sewn shut
to conserve tears, kidneys like petrified wood,
a list of bleak outcomes—blindness, lymphoma.
This healer offers me yellow fever pills
as if they would juice up my rasping cunt
or stop my teeth from rattling like castanets.

"Somebody's Knocking"

A Prednisone song

I'm alone when the bell chimes late at night.
I should know better, but I open the door.
He slouches in the porch light, wearing
tight jeans slung over hard hips, a grin
that lights a fire where I sit.
"Candy, little girl?" He winks, opens
a meaty fist. Tiny pills the color
of robins' eggs shine against
his callused palm, just the right
size to go down easy. I want
to shake my head and close the door
but fever burns under my lids, joints
throb and my gut begs for relief.
"We can fly," he says, running
a fingertip up my arm. I lean into him,
remember how the engine-revving rush
whisks away bellyaches, bone pain,
blood from all the wrong places
and lick my dry lips. "You can only
stay a little while," I finally say.

The Truth about Travel

Skipping time zones leaves me with gritty eyes
and a headache. I know too much about lumpy
hotel beds, foreigners who refuse to speak English,
long hours in a car or bus, picture-book scenery
whizzing by while I wish for a bathroom, a chance
to stretch, somebody new to talk to over dinner.
Then there's the food—greasy pub fare, bloodwurst
or fried meat of unknown origin. Only the memories
make it worthwhile. Standing at the kitchen sink,
for a moment I hear again jazz in a Prague square,
stroll down a certain waterfront alley in Cannes,
or dance the polka on a snowy night near Salzburg.

Now I'm dizzy and weak, like the time that my head
swam in a Devon farmhouse after pub hopping,
when I mistook a cow for a woman moaning in sex.
Rising from the commode where I've knelt all night,
I recall a week of cramps in a Rhine village and a doctor
only too glad to take my American cash. In the mirror
my skin gleams with a damp sheen, like the moss
on ancient stone walls between Yorkshire fields,
the mortar of my health as crumbling as those walls.
In the bathroom mirror my face wears the waxy
translucence of a cryptal effigy in Westminster Abbey
and I wonder why I ever wanted to leave home.

The Rehearsal

I hate to cook, yet I make a feast of fresh vegetables—
creamed corn, fried okra, green beans, ripe tomatoes—
to eat with buttery corn sticks. "It's ready," I say,
and the world goes blank. My husband calls the doctor,
tells him I'm acting like a drunk trying to pass for sober.
On the way to the hospital where I work, twin cars
whiz in double lanes. My vision clears, but some
silly woman's jabber falls out of my mouth. "A clot
on the brain stem," the doctor says. Knowing I can
become a vegetable like those on my table, I giggle
while the internist grills me about secret drinking.

My good sense has gone on vacation. It's as if
I've forgotten my grandmother Annie, her dread
of stroke, I fold my arms, let them slide me,
who can hardly breathe in subways, into a tube
for an MRI. I lie still for a doctor to shove a hose
down my throat to look for clots lurking in my heart.
The lab reports bleeding time in the danger zone,
yet I, the nurse, only ask if I got to eat any
of the corn, the beans. The next day the doctor yanks
the IV, declares me out of danger. On the ride home
I fear a wreck, the street awash with my blood.

The next two weeks, I struggle with simple words,
run red lights, cut up credit cards for no reason
until the mist clears, and, like Annie, I know terror.

Going Steady

Diseases are often named for the doctors
who first catalogue their symptoms.

What woman hasn't imagined being
in bed with more than one man?
But a good girl, long married, I was never
into the kinky stuff. Suddenly my fantasy
comes true: three new guys share me.
If it were high school, I would wear
a senior ring caked with wax,
a letterman's jacket, sleeves rolled up,
a fraternity pin over my left tit.
My new lovers, doctors all—
Wouldn't my mother be proud?
—hardly let me get out of bed.
These sexy seducers leave brands
like whisker burns and sucking kisses.

Dr. Sjögren, that charming Swede,
likes to talk nasty, "Head case, long
in the tooth, dry as a bone."
Dr. Reynaud, French to the core,
kisses my lilac fingertips, navy nail beds,
murmuring, *"Froid hands, chaud heart."*
Dr. Crohn, that plain-speaking American,
thinks foreplay is whispers of stomach
in knots, gut feeling, pain in the ass.
These men don't have a jealous bone.
I can still flirt with guys in hard hats
sporting tattoos on rocky biceps.
Lefty Lupus says my skin rash turns him on.
His pal, Slammo Sclera D., would like
to lick my smooth knuckles, but for once
I'm too exhausted to think about sex.

Big Sky Country

In Atlanta on Ozone Alert Days, when heat
shimmers on asphalt and buildings wear
a skim-milk haze, I conjure the Montana
of summer vacations, warm days,
fireside nights. Outside of Red Lodge,
I know how prairie grass waves,
a woman's hair in water, the silver-tipped
Beartooth Range rises, offering valley vistas.
In Luther, a dozen mailboxes cluster,
not a house in sight, and in Bear Creek
a bar draws pickups like birds to a feeder.
I watched Friday-night drinkers bet
paychecks on piglets scampering out back
around a dirt oval while the barkeep tells us
how in winter, iguanas race between tables.

I'm ready to turn my car northwest.
But then I think winter, arctic cold,
snowy quiet, scuttling lizards underfoot.
It's too much like life since I gave up
my nursing job and became a patient,
since my strength dribbled down to
afternoon naps. Friends say I have it made.
They don't know hours unreel, endless prairie.
Instead of lacing on boots to tackle
a rocky path, I face worse dangers than rattlers,
a stray grizzly—poison pills, drifting clots,
sluggard kidneys, a gut at war with itself.
I can't tell them this trek I didn't choose
looms steeper than any wilderness trail.

Body Shop

I clock in at dawn to enter rooms
stinking of old blood, much-breathed air.
Patients sprawl on beds like stalled cars,
their bodies revealing secrets no one
wants to know: tired cupid bows of urethra,
dimpled epidermal moonscapes, leering
new mouths carved by surgeons.
Safe in my scrubs, I catalog symptoms,
tell smiling lies, stroke patients' arms
to rub them in. My hands move with
precision, bandaging proud flesh,
programming pumps, mainlining drugs.
Talking to heads, working on bodies.

Patients' stories flatten into blips
on a screen, ink smears in a chart,
puzzle pieces to fit into a pattern.
Until now I could hang up my scrubs
and clock out, but I've become
one of them—symptoms, syndromes,
a prognosis. My charges complain
of chilled fingers, the breaks I take
to swallow pills. Medical Records keeps
a growing folder under my name,
a rap sheet of my body's convictions,
I plead my case to the bored nurse
I am, but she shrugs. She's seen it all.

The Greedy Dead

I buried Mother twenty-five years ago,
but she still whispers: *"Stand up straight,*
smile, don't let men know you're smart."
My sister escaped, but I stayed—a confessor
for Mother's sins, a record keeper of small
slights, a protester to suicide schemes.
But I couldn't save her. On her sixtieth
birthday she wore lace to a solo party.
Instead of cake, she ate red jelly sleepers.

After so many years I think myself safe
from those heirloom pearls of gloom.
Yet, three months before I would turn
sixty, I lie in the hospital, my bone
marrow on strike, lungs swampy, my heart
chugging like a Model T. My sister
calls me: "Today is Mother's birthday.
Do you think she is reaching for you?"

I think how Mother would sit beside me,
my hand curled in hers, as she dumped
her problems, smothering me under the weight,
then grin. "Don't worry about me."
Outside my window a magnolia blooms.
I stare at petals as white as her Ipana smile.
Mother's hand beckons among glossy leaves,
but I won't be the good daughter again.

Saying Thank You

A Southerner, I thought I knew
good manners—you first, please this,
thank you that. So over tea at an inn,
I ask a woman about herself.
"New York is home, but I came back
for my sick mother." Cancer, it always
comes down to that, or so I had thought.
Now I knew worse terrors—bad doctors,
bungling nurses, nearly dying for no reason.

From porch rockers we look out at
mountains gaudy with fall leaves.
"I climbed Mount LeConte last year.
Now I'm barely walking." I describe
transfusions by the quart, boggy lungs,
marrow gone on strike, a daughter who
stood guard like a pit bull, checking on
nurses, tracking monitors, grilling doctors.

"My mother died six months ago.
What hurt was how she thanked me—
for every little act." Remembering how
I, too, had thanked my daughter when
she mothered me, I say, "She knew."
Thank you was all I had left to give.
The words slipped out with every breath,
no longer manners, but an act like prayer.

The Safe Zone

It's like when you were ten, and your mother calls
and calls for you to come in from a game of tag just
as the lightening bugs begin to flash, and her voice
gets that sawtooth edge you know means trouble.
It's when you run inside and flop down on the couch.
After she's done fussing and the crease between
her brows erases, she undoes your stubby braids,
pulling her fingers through your hair, a tingle
like dancing fairies that makes your eyes fall shut.

Or it's like that trip to Prague, all night knotted
in a plane seat, an hour of riding over bumpy roads
with a driver who doesn't know a word of English
as you hug your bag with money and passport,
knowing that if you disappeared now, no one
could find you. It's after you pay the driver the sum
he writes on a slip of paper, even if it's too much,
so he will hand you the key. When you lock the door
and your head hits the pillow, the dreams start
while your eyes are still open, and you can let go
of the thick meringue pressing on your brain.

Except this time you're curled in a hospital bed,
the air conditioning on your backside, the only air
moving, certainly not in your lungs, that festering
mucous swamp, and you pant like a hound in July.
You don't dare sleep: sloppy nurses could bring
germs to finish you off or flood your heart with
the IV's two-step drip, the blood's thick crawl.
It's this new nurse, just when you've given up.
It's her stare over a stethoscope as she nods in time
to your stuttering pulse, reads the news in your
lungs' wet-paper wheeze. At last you can rest,
your lids drooping like sheets hung out in the rain.

Doppelgänger

I'm here to tell you it's not that easy being
two people at once. The nurse that I am nods,
noting symptoms. Yes, bone marrow suppression,
pneumonia, left ventricular hypertrophy
indicate a poor prognosis. As the patient,
short of breath, head split by bolts of pain,
I push the call button, count minutes until
a frazzled woman with a clipboard rushes in,
only to wait again for the pill, the relief.
The other nurses, the doctors, know I'm
a member of the club. We talk critical
platelet counts, rocketing hypertension.
Alone, I dial the automated report number.
"Webster, Anne: today's chest film shows
increased infiltrates of pneumonia."
Pus boils in needle sticks; my fever spikes.
Is this the fatal infection? I've seen it all
too many times to think I should be spared.
Yet the woman that is me weeps for the man
she would leave, the shining years left, for
grandchildren who will grow up without her,
even as the nurse in me notes vital signs, tallies
figures in the chart, numbers in the red zone.

ACKNOWLEDGMENTS

Grateful acknowledgment is made to the editors of the following publications, in which these poems or versions of these poems first appeared:

Cedar Hills Review: the women's issue: "Two Girls Named Alice"; *Dekalb Literary Arts Journal*: "Burial"; *Georgia State University Review*: "Intensive Care"; *Mediphors, A Literary Journal of the Health Professions*: "True Colors"; *Nebo, A Literary Journal*: "My Mentor"; *The New York Quarterly*: "A History of Nursing"; *Off P'tree: Atlanta's Magazine of Arts and Entertainment*: "How Does Your Garden Grow?"; *Piedmont Literary Review*: "Modern Nursing"; *Phantasm*: "The Exhibitionist"; *Southern Poetry Review*: "Sunday Prayer"; *Sunstone Review*: "My Father's War"; *The White Crow*: "Who Will Mother the Mothers?"

"Acquittal" and "Mother & Daddy in Sepia" from *O, Georgia! A Collection of Georgia's Newest and Most Promising Writers*, Humpus Bumpus Press (1999).

"Doppelgänger" from *Stories of Illness and Healing: Women Write Their Bodies*, Kent State University Press (2007).

"Doppelgänger" and "Stuff I Learned in Nursing School" from *Intensive Care: More Poems and Prose by Nurses*, University of Iowa Press (2003).

"Going Steady," "The House on Bolton Road," "True Colors," and "The Woman My Husband Should Have Married" from The *Poetry of Nursing: Poems and Commentary of Leading Nurse Poets*, reprinted with the permission of Kent State University Press (2006).

"Mein Liebes Deutschland" from *Vacations: The Good, the Bad, and the Ugly*, Outrider Press (2006).

"My Father's War" also appeared in *Ethic American Woman: Problems, Protests, Lifestyle*, Kendall/Hunt Publishing (1978).

"Dry Drowning" appears in *Rattle, Poetry for the 21st Century*, Volume 13, Number 2, Winter 2007.

A Call to Nursing, Kaplan Publishing, for Spring 2009 release: "Sondercommando," "The Safe Zone," and "Slow Night in the ER".

90

92

LaVergne, TN USA
18 August 2009
155050LV00014B/48/P

9 781933 483177